PERFECT HEALTH & REVERSE AGING

MASTERCLASS ON DIET, WORKOUT, LIFE BALANCE, TOTAL HEALTH

Table of Contents

WHY A COURSE ON PERFECT HEALTH & REVERSING AGING?

- Because we can - And – if we can increase the quality of our life as well – we should try

- People are living longer and have the means to do so

- Quality of life is everything at any age – especially as we age

- Science has taught us how to live optimally, healthfully, happily

- Let's explore the possibilities and see what works for you and I

- Let's get and stay healthy consciously and with purpose & meaning

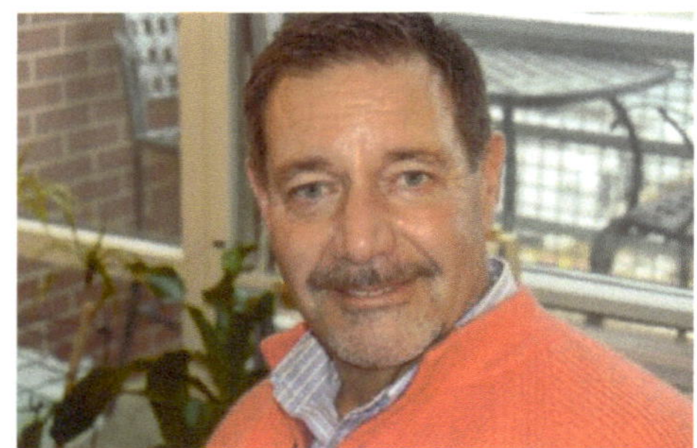

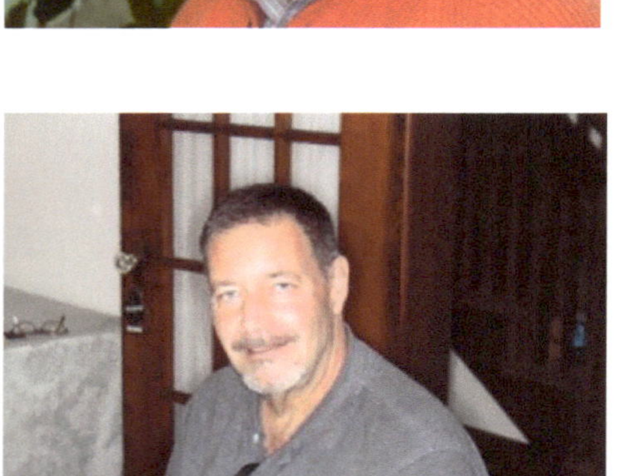

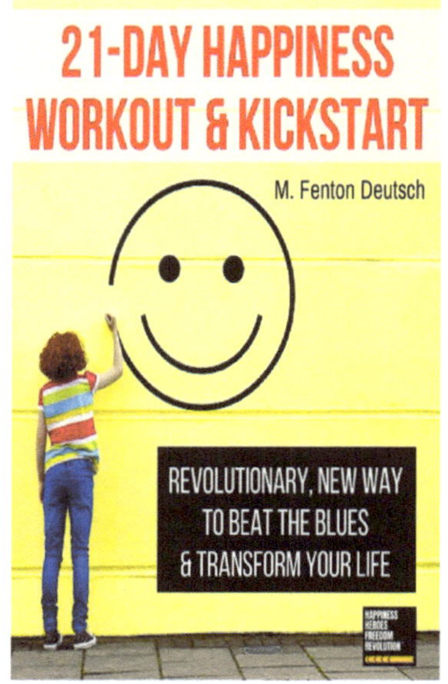

21-DAY HAPPINESS
WORKOUT & KICKSTART
M. Fenton Deutsch
REVOLUTIONARY, NEW WAY
TO BEAT THE BLUES
& TRANSFORM YOUR LIFE

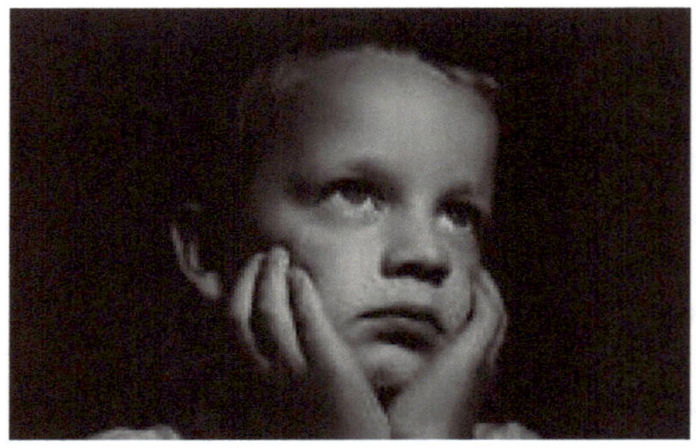

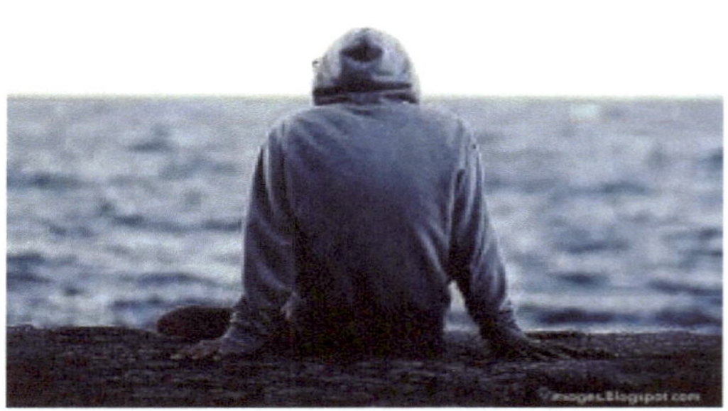

IS THERE A FOUNTAIN OF YOUTH TODAY?

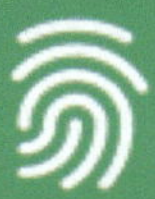

Much has been written about Ponce de Leon, who claimed the Native Indians told him such a drinking and bathing fountain could be found in Bimini –off the coast of Florida.

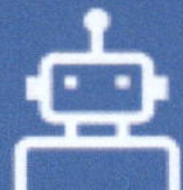

The ancients have always talked about immortality – and some say that it lies somewhere in Ethopia.

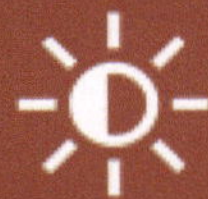

No matter, science and quantum physics have finally caught up with spirituality and entrepreneurship.

There is much we can learn and practice from the experts – so have fun!

THE WHOLE TRUTH?

- With ever-increasing advances in science and medicine, people are living longer, and this trend towards healthy aging is likely to continue

- Want to live as long as possible, healthy, wealthy, and wise?

- Focus on changing the way and what you eat, exercise, learn to manage stress, fortify your immune system to fight disease, focus on living your life with and on purpose, and with meaning, focus on great experiences shared in healthy, long-lasting relationships, focus on happiness before success, and live well into old age

- Study the habits, rituals, routines, and lifestyles of Highly Happy People, Healthy People, Long-Living people and cultures

- Learn how to practice the science of longevity: Diet, Nutrition, Exercise, Lifestyle, Stress Management, Focus on Happiness & Quality of Life

- Learn how to find our true "Fountain of Youth" that is already inside of us – Our Spiritual Natures

- Learn how to marry our insides with our outsides for as along and happily as possible

STUDY BLUE ZONES

- "Inspired by the world's longest-lived cultures, Blue Zones claims to help you live longer, better

- Reverse Engineering Longevity: Life expectancy of an American born today averages 78.2 years. But this year, over 70,000 Americans have reached their 100th birthday. What are they doing that the average American isn't? To answer the question, we teamed up with National Geographic to find the world's longest-lived people and study them. We knew most of the answers lied within their lifestyle and environment (The Danish Twin Study established that only about 20% of how long the average person lives is determined by genes). Then we worked with a team of demographers to find pockets of people around the world with the highest life expectancy, or with the highest proportions of people who reach age 100.

- We found five places that met our criteria:

- Barbagia region of Sardinia – Mountainous highlands of inner Sardinia with the world's highest concentration of male centenarians.

- Ikaria, Greece – Aegean Island with one of the world's lowest rates of middle age mortality and the lowest rates of dementia.

- Nicoya Peninsula, Costa Rica – World's lowest rates of middle age mortality, second highest concentration of male centenarians.

- Seventh Day Adventists – Highest concentration is around Loma Linda, California. They live 10 years longer than their North American counterparts.

- Okinawa, Japan – Females over 70 are the longest-lived population in the world.

- Source: Bluezones.com Power 9® Reverse Engineering Longevity By Dan Buettner : Same Source & Atribution for Next 9 Slides

- Take this Longevity Quiz to establish your baseline: https://apps.bluezones.com/en/vitality/background

Blue Zones assembled a team of medical researchers, anthropologists, demographers, and epidemiologists to search for evidence-based common denominators among all places. We found nine.

1. 1. Move Naturally

2. 2. Purpose

3. 3. Down Shift

4. 4. 80% Rule

5. 5. Plant Slant

6. 8. Loved Ones First

7. 9. Right Tribe

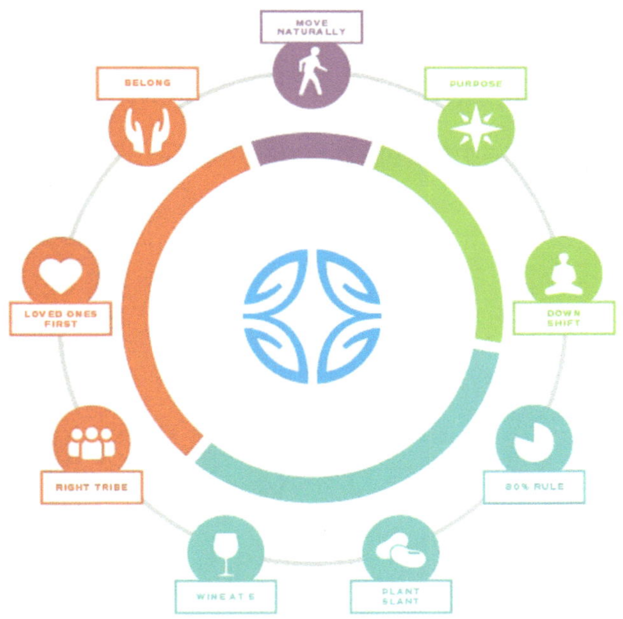

- The world's longest-lived people don't pump iron, run marathons or join gyms. Instead, they live in environments that constantly nudge them into moving without thinking about it. They grow gardens and don't have mechanical conveniences for house and yard work.

The Okinawans call it "Ikigai" and the Nicoyans call it "plan de vida;" for both it translates to "why I wake up in the morning." Knowing your sense of purpose is worth up to seven years of extra life expectancy

3. DOWN SHIFT

Even people in the Blue Zones experience stress. Stress leads to chronic inflammation, associated with every major age-related disease. What the world's longest-lived people have that we don't are routines to shed that stress. Okinawans take a few moments each day to remember their ancestors, Adventists pray, Ikarians take a nap and Sardinians do happy hour.

"Hara hachi bu" – the Okinawan, 2500-year old Confucian mantra said before meals reminds them to stop eating when their stomachs are 80 percent full. The 20% gap between not being hungry and feeling full could be the difference between losing weight or gaining it. People in the Blue Zones eat their smallest meal in the late afternoon or early evening and then they don't eat any more the rest of the day.

5. PLANT SLANT

Beans, including fava, black, soy and lentils, are the cornerstone of most centenarian diets. Meat—mostly pork—is eaten on average only five times per month. Serving sizes are 3-4 oz., about the size of a deck of cards.

People in all Blue Zones (except Adventists) drink alcohol moderately and regularly. Moderate drinkers outlive non-drinkers. The trick is to drink 1-2 glasses per day (preferably Sardinian Cannonau wine), with friends and/or with food. And no, you can't save up all week and have 14 drinks on Saturday.

7. BELONG-BELIEVE

All but five of the 263 centenarians we interviewed belonged to some faith-based community. Denomination doesn't seem to matter. Research shows that attending faith-based services four times per month will add 4-14 years of life expectancy.

8. LOVED ONES FIRST

Successful centenarians in the Blue Zones put their families first. This means keeping aging parents and grandparents nearby or in the home (It lowers disease and mortality rates of children in the home too.). They commit to a life partner (which can add up to 3 years of life expectancy) and invest in their children with time and love (They'll be more likely to care for you when the time comes).

- The world's longest lived people chose—or were born into—social circles that supported healthy behaviors, Okinawans created "moais"–groups of five friends that committed to each other for life. Research from the Framingham Studies shows that smoking, obesity, happiness, and even loneliness are contagious. So the social networks of long-lived people have favorably shaped their health behaviors.

- To make it to age 100, you have to have won the genetic lottery. But most of us have the capacity to make it well into our early 90's and largely without chronic disease. As the Adventists demonstrate, the average person's life expectancy could increase by 10-12 years by adopting a Blue Zones lifestyle.

- A number of different measures contribute to the average overall happiness of any given country, including GDP per capita, life expectancy, freedom to make life choices, and even overall generosity and social support. These are the countries (they are not in chronological order) ranked top 20 by 2014 Legatum Prosperity Index.

- 1. Finland, 2. Norway, 3. Denmark, 4. Iceland, 5. Switzerland, 6. The Netherlands, 7. Canada, 8. New Zealand, 9. Sweden, 10. Australia...18. U.S. 19. United Kingdom

- Location plays a hand in how bright or gloomy our days are. For years, researchers have studied the science of happiness and found that its key ingredients include a positive mental state, healthy body, strong social connections, job satisfaction and financial well-being.

- Sioux Falls, SD

- Lincoln, NE

- Olathe, KS

- Overland Park, KS

- Omaha, NE

- Boise City, ID

- Lexington, KY

- Cary, NC

- Madison, WI

- Wichita, KS

- Source: https://www.theladders.com/career-advice/these-are-the-top-10-happiest-cities-in-america-for-2018

THE 10 CITIES WITH THE BEST QUALITY OF LIFE IN THE WORLD

- Source: Business Insider: Every year Mercer, one of the world's largest HR consultancy firms, releases its Quality of Living Index, which looks at which cities provide the best quality of life. The ranking is one of the most comprehensive of its kind and is carried out annually to help multinational companies and other employers to compensate employees fairly when placing them on international assignments, according to Mercer.

- London and New York do not make it anywhere near the top of the list.

- 1.Vienna-Austria 2.Zurich-Switzerland 3.Auckland,NZ/Munich-Germany,5.Vancouver, Canada, 6. Dusseldorf, Germany, 7. Frankfurt, Germany, 8. Geneva, Switzerland, 9. Copenhagen, Denmark, Basel, Switzerland

- A heart-healthy diet is one that includes:

- Fruits and vegetables.

- Whole grains.

- Low-fat dairy products like yogurt and cheese.

- Skinless poultry.

- Lots of fish.

- Nuts and beans.

- Non-tropical vegetable oils (olive, corn, peanut, and safflower oils)

- Source: Web MD- https://www.webmd.com/healthy-aging/features/longevity-foods#1

- Blue Zone Diet:

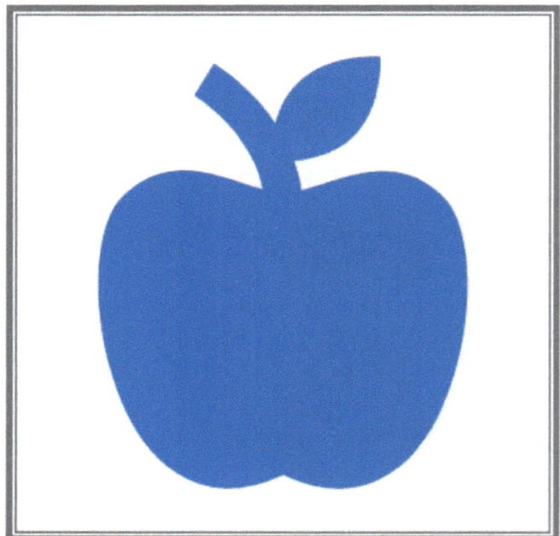

BLUE ZONE DIET

For a long life and better health, try boosting your intake of foods that people living in Blue Zones have in their diet. A concept developed by National Geographic Fellow and author Dan Buettner, Blue Zones are areas across the globe where people tend to live the longest and have remarkably low rates of heart disease, cancer, diabetes, and obesity.

Although food choices vary from region to region,Blue Zone diets are primarily plant-based, with as much as 95 percent of daily food intake coming from vegetables,fruits,grains,and legumes. People in Blue Zones typically avoid meat and dairy, as well as sugary foods and beverages.

Source: Bluezone.com and Verywellhealth https://www.verywellhealth.com/blue-zone-diet-foods-4159314

- From chickpeas to lentils, legumes are a vital component of all Blue Zone diets. Loaded with fiber and known for their heart-healthy effects, legumes also serve as a top source of protein, complex carbohydrates, and a variety of vitamins and minerals.

- Whether you prefer pinto beans or black-eyed peas, aim for at least a half-cup of legumes each day. Ideal for any meal, legumes make a great addition to salads, soups and stews, and many veggie-based recipes. "If you want to make a three-bean chili for dinner, use dry beans and soak them, cooking them with your own spices and fresh veggies," recommends registered dietician Maya Feller, owner of Maya Feller Nutrition.

DARK LEAFY GREENS

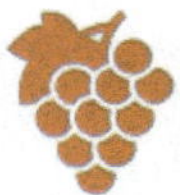

- While vegetables of all kinds abound in each Blue Zone diet, dark leafy greens like kale, spinach, and Swiss chard are especially prized. One of the most nutrient-dense types of veggies, dark leafy greens contain several vitamins with powerful antioxidant properties, including vitamin A and vitamin C.

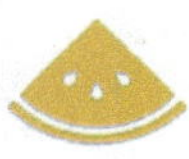

- When shopping for any kind of veggie, remember that people in Blue Zones generally consume locally grown, organically farmed vegetables.

Like legumes, nuts are packed with protein, vitamins, and minerals. They also supply heart-healthy unsaturated fats, with some research suggesting that including nuts in your diet may help reduce your cholesterol levels (and, in turn, stave off cardiovascular disease).

"Nuts are a high-fiber food," says Feller. "Almonds, for instance, provide about 3.5 grams of fiber in a one-ounce serving." For healthier snacking, borrow a habit from Blue Zone residents and try a handful of almonds, walnuts, pistachios, cashews, or Brazil nuts.

- A staple of Blue Zone diets, olive oil offers a wealth of health-enhancing fatty acids, antioxidants, and compounds such as oleuropein (a chemical found to curb inflammation).

- Many studies have shown that olive oil may improve heart health in a number of ways, such as by keeping cholesterol and blood pressure in check. What's more, emerging research indicates that olive oil could help protect against conditions like Alzheimer's disease and diabetes.

- Select the extra-virgin variety of olive oil as often as possible, and use your oil for cooking and in salads and vegetable dishes. Olive oil is sensitive to light and heat, so be sure to store it in a cool, dark area like a kitchen cabinet.

- When it comes to whole grains, those in Blue Zones often choose oats. One of the least processed forms of oats, steel-cut oats make for a high-fiber and incredibly filling breakfast option.

- Although they're perhaps best-known for their cholesterol-lowering power, oats may also provide plenty of other health benefits. For instance, recent research has determined that oats may thwart weight gain, fight diabetes, and prevent hardening of the arteries.

- "Oats are known for their fiber content, but they also provide plant-based protein," says Feller. "Oatmeal made with 1/4 cup of steel cut oats provides 7 grams of protein."

BLUEBERRIES

- Fresh fruit is the go-to sweet treat for many people living in Blue Zones. While most any type of fruit can make for a healthy dessert or snack, foods such as blueberries may offer bonus benefits. For example, recent studies have demonstrated that blueberries may help shield your brain health as you age, and fend off heart disease by improving blood pressure control.

- For other Blue Zone-friendly but sweet-tooth-satisfying eats, look to such fruits as papayas, pineapples, bananas, and strawberries.

BARLEY

- Another whole grain favored in Blue Zones, barley may possess cholesterol-lowering properties similar to those of oats, according to a study recently published in the European Journal of Clinical Nutrition. Barley also delivers essential amino acids, as well as compounds that may help stimulate digestion.

To get your fill of barley, try adding this whole grain to soups or consuming it as a hot cereal.

- These anti-aging foods will help you eat your way to a longer life expectancy. Add these delicious foods into your daily diet and you will be decreasing your risk for illnesses and age-related problems. Just pick one or two to add in each week.

- have to be one of the most delicious foods out there. Mix up a little guacamole or slice a few up on your salad for an anti-aging treat. Avocados are one of the best foods around for anti-aging and longevity. Why? First of all, they are delicious. But more importantly, avocados are filled with healthy fats and other nutrients to help your body live longer and work better.

- Avocados

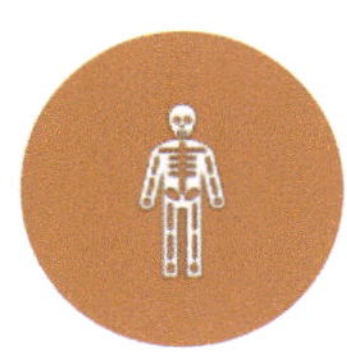

- Source: Verywellhealth-By Mark Stibich, PhD

WALNUTS

- Walnuts are the perfect snack for anti-aging. They give you protein and omega-3s in a safe, convenient form. Eat a handful every day. Walnuts are a great anti-aging food because of the amount of omega-3s in just a handful. These omega-3 fatty acids are real longevity tools. They prevent dementia and keep your brain young while fighting off heart disease by improving your cholesterol. Make walnuts part of your day, every day.

- Eating your vegetables for anti-aging may not seem like interesting advice, but the impact of eating enough vegetables on your life expectancy is extreme. Vegetables are a great source of nutrients and antioxidants. Not only that, but vegetables also help you lose weight. Eat five to nine servings every day to help your body make repairs and live longer.

- Our bodies need water to fight off aging and damage. Drink lots of water every day to keep your body functioning well. Water is a multi-billion dollar industry. There are many claims that water can be healthy and even "detox" your body. Most of these claims are not fully backed by research. However, it seems obvious that drinking lots of water is a good thing, even if it is only because you are not drinking other sugary beverages.

- The fact that chocolate has anti-aging properties is proof that the universe is a kind and loving place. Eat chocolate (not too much) for anti-aging benefits. Chocolate is one of the world's favorite foods. Recent research shows that eating moderate amounts of dark chocolate also brings health benefits to your heart. The antioxidants in dark chocolate protect your heart against aging, damage, and heart disease.

- For an anti-aging dessert, have a bowl full of berries. Pack in those vitamins and avoid sugary alternatives. Berries are a great source of antioxidants and other nutrients. Eat more strawberries, blueberries, and blackberries to help with anti-aging and longevity. Not only do berries fight free radicals that cause damage to your body, they also provide other essential nutrients. Work berries into your weekly diet.

RED WINE

- Good news! Red wine has properties to make you younger. Just a glass or two a day has amazing anti-aging benefits. Red wine has been reported to have a multitude of health benefits. Over 400 scientific studies support some benefit to red wine. Studies giving mice incredibly amounts of some of the components of red wine show tremendous benefits in protecting against unhealthy eating habits.

- Green tea is an ancient drink for good health and longevity. The antioxidant benefits of daily consumption of green tea are well known. A little drink of green tea a couple of times a day could do wonders for your life expectancy. Switching green tea for sodas in the afternoon would have multiple benefits.

MELONS

- Melons are delicious. They are also a great source of a wide range of vitamins. Eat a different kind of melon every week for excellent health benefits. Melons are a delicious source of vitamins and other nutrients. Watermelons and cantaloupe are easy-to-find and inexpensive sources of great anti-aging foods. Add melons to your daily foods for a big healthy boost to your diet.

- eart will love the healthy, fat-free protein, and other anti aging properties of beans. Beans are a great anti-aging and longevity food. They provide healthy protein without all the fat that you find in animal products. Beans also provide a big supply of antioxidants that prevent damage by free radicals. Work beans into your weekly menu for their anti-aging properties.

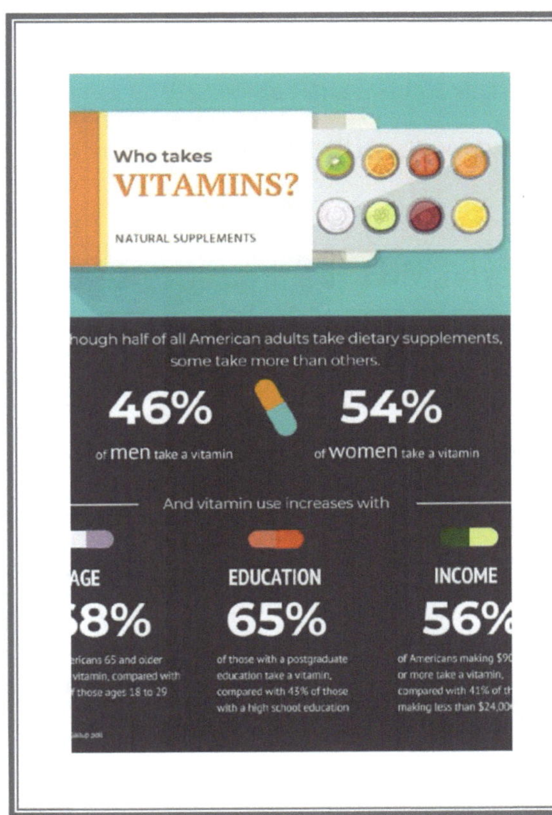

- Older Americans Hooked on Vitamins Even Though Little Evidence They Work

- There's no conclusive evidence that dietary supplements prevent chronic disease in the average American, Manson said. And while a handful of vitamin and mineral studies have had positive results, those findings haven't been strong enough to recommend supplements to the general U.S. public, she said.

- Eat GREAT food, and forget about supplements unless advised by doctors' orders

BEST LONGEVITY, HEALTHY DIETS

- The nutritarian diet is an eating pattern created by Dr. Joel Fuhrman initially published in his top-selling 2003 diet book Eat to Live. The diet is vegan, gluten-free, low in sodium, and low in fat https://www.youtube.com/watch?v=E4katnfHzXA

- Part of "undo it," The Ornish diet is a type of vegetarian diet that can reverse the symptoms of heart disease. … "On the Ornish diet, people eat beans, legumes, fruits, grains and vegetables," said Dr. Martin. "You can also eat some low-fat and nonfat dairy products like milk, cheese and yogurt. https://www.google.com/search?ei=aD71XlfwJqqd_QaD_q5I&q=dean+ornish+ted+talk&oq=dean+or&gs_l=psy-ab.1.1.0j0i67j0l8.12242.15575..18380...1.0..0.99.652.8......0....1..gws-wiz.....6..0i71j35i39j0i131j0i10i67j0i3.uMvB24AoPgk

- https://health.usnews.com/best-diet/best-healthy-eating-diets

- https://www.webmd.com/healthy-aging/features/longevity-foods#1

- Centenarians in the "Blue Zones" areas live in environments that nudge them to move naturally every twenty minutes, rather than separating fitness into a different part of their day. It's built into their lifestyles subconsciously. Their habits may make you want to abandon fitness altogether.

- BUT...

- Plan a smarter week of workouts to give your routine—and results—a major boost. With benefits like better quality sleep, a boost in brainpower, and increased levels of happiness, it's no wonder why exercise is a major part of your daily routine. The fact that you're getting up and out is a win in itself, but science and experts agree: there are loads of benefits to diversifying your workouts, especially if you want to avoid injury.

- "Variety is the spice of fitness," says Adam Rosante, celebrity strength and nutrition coach. "One of the surest ways to hit a plateau is to do the same workout over and over."

- Monday: Upper-body strength training (45 to 60 minutes)

- Tuesday: Lower-body strength training (30 to 60 minutes)

- Wednesday: Yoga or a low-impact activity like barre, light cycling, or swimming (30 to 60 minutes)

- Thursday: HIIT (High Impact Interval Training (20 minutes)

- Friday: Total-body strength training (30 to 60 minutes)

- Saturday: Steady-state cardio (running or cycling for as long as feels comfortable for you)

- Sunday: Rest (Don't forget to foam roll and stretch!)

- Source: Shape   https://www.shape.com/fitness/training-plans/perfectly-balanced-week-workouts

- For us older folk, combine aerobic (walking, running, bicycle, spin with yoga/stretch and strength training – mostly light weights and cross fit. Join a class, hire a trainer, or get some great videos. Also, dance, swim, play sports anywhere, stretch before and after working out. Drink lots of water (8 glasses or ½ gallon/day). Stay away from hard liquor and clearly no drugs or anything in an abusive manner. If you need help, get it!

- If you're not going to move to blue zones or best countries, cities or towns to live in, try to build a sustainable routine to manage stress:

- The 7 Best Workouts for Stress ReliefEveryone gets stressed out. It's a normal part of life – but that doesn't mean you should just deal with it! There are many techniques, activities, and therapies that can help relieve stress, but exercise just might be the most beneficial way to naturally reduce stress.

- Why? Physical activity reduces cortisol levels (your body's stress hormone). Getting active and breaking a sweat causes your body to produce endorphins, which help your body and mind relax. You can expect better sleep, a clear mind, and an improved mood thanks to a stress-relieving workout session. Yoga,

- Tai Chi, Gardening, Kickboxing, Dancing, Outdoor Activity,

- Source: https://www.huffpost.com/entry/the-7-best-workouts-for-stress-relief_b_5 91b5165e4b03e1c81b00987   https://www.youtube.com/watch?v=hBP-YBX597s

- Destress yourself by taking non-essential things off your To-Do list, give yourself time in between tasks, focus on mindfulness and presence for the things you are doing

- Have Less by decluttering and getting rid of non-essential, non-purposeful things in your house, bedroom kitchen, closets, and at work.

- 10 steps for decluttering the Marie Kondo way

- Declutter BEFORE organizing. …

- Take photos of your spaces before you begin. …

- Start the tidying up process with clothes first. …

- Hold each item in your hands, and ask yourself, "Does this item bring me joy?" …

- Before getting rid of an item, hold it and say, "Thank you" …

- Fold clothes the Marie Kondo way. …

- Tidy sentimental items last.

- https://www.mother.ly/news/10-steps-for-decluttering-the-marie-kondo-way

- Time Management: Work Smarter, Not Harder: Complete most important tasks first. …Learn to say "no". …Sleep at least 7-8 hours. …Devote your entire focus to the task at hand. …Get an early start. …Don't allow unimportant details to drag you down. …Turn key tasks into habits. Source: https://www.creativitypost.com/create/work_smarter_not_harder_21_time_management_tips_to_hack_productivity

- How to Set Goals & Priorities: Choose the right goals. Try to find the middle ground between aiming too high and not high enough. …Make it formal. Writing down the goal will make it official and will add to your sense of commitment. …Devise a plan. This is vital in making the goal a reality. …Stick to it, but stay flexible. …Regularly reassess. Source: https://psychcentral.com/lib/top-tips-for-setting-goals-and-priorities/

- Morning Rituals:

- What is Self-Love?

- In short, self-love is the forgiveness, acceptance, and respect for who you are deep down – all your beautiful and hideous parts included. When you love yourself, you take care of yourself, you honor your limitations, you listen to your needs and you respect your dreams enough to act on them. When you love yourself, your happiness, health, and fulfillment are all of supreme importance because you realize that without loving yourself, you will never be able to genuinely love others. Source: LonerWolf.com

- How to Love Others: Love as Patience, Love as Kindness, Love as delight in others' successes, Love as humility, Love as empathy. Source: tiny buddha, Joel Almeida - https://tinybuddha.com/blog/5-ways-show-love-others-yourself/

- https://www.google.com/w&q=ted+talks%2Chow+to+love+yourself+and+others&oq=ted+talks%2Chow+to+love+yourself+and+others&gs_l=psy-ab.3..33i22i29i30.4141.10404..10508...0.0..2.252.6477.0j37j3......0....1..gws-wiz.......0i71j35i39j0i131i67j0i131j0i67j0j0i20i263j0i22i30j33i299j33i160.S_p5Nhd4WnY#kpvalbx=1

- https://www.youtube.com/watch?v=vMeEKBaiPbg

- Click on and practice these amazing resources:

- https://www.nytimes.com/guides/well/how-to-meditate

- https://www.nytimes.com/guides/well/be-more-mindful-at-work

- https://www.nytimes.com/guides/well/activity/basic-mindfulness-meditation

- https://www.youtube.com/watch?v=TJhvfvDzwE0

- https://www.youtube.com/watch?v=V4zhQ3M892E

- https://www.youtube.com/watch?v=qUYRYRvr5G8

DEVELOP A MORNING RITUAL AND ROUTINE

- CREATE YOUR OWN SIMPLE AND EFFECTIVE MORNING RITUAL: Take out a journal, notepad, text document, or Google Keep note. Ask yourself what you need to do each moment in the morning to stop just going through the motions and create the purpose-filled, joyful, simple life you desire. Then write it down along with about how much time each step should take. Ask anyone involved if they can support you in creating this morning ritual, being sure to tell them how the whole household will benefit. Post a reminder by your bed so that tomorrow morning you can remember to begin the new habit of doing your morning ritual upon waking every day.

- Resources: https://www.inc.com/bryan-adams/6-celebrity-morning-rituals-to-help-you-kick-ass.html My personal favorite: https://www.youtube.com/watch?v=aTlqTNje7q

- https://www.youtube.com/watch?v=EXbUFgqjMdk

- Ihttps://www.youtube.com/watch?v=Kvs-_22lwjA&t=140s

BUILD YOUR HAPPINESS ARCHITECTURE

- 5 Ways to Turn Happiness Into An Advantage (Shawn Achor The Happiness Advantage) Reversing the formula for happiness and success. It's hard to find happiness after success if the goalposts of success keep changing. Do this for at least 21-days – enough time to form new habits.

- 1. Write down three new things you are grateful for each day into a blank word document..Journal. Research shows this will significantly improve your optimism even 6 months later, and raises your success rates significantly.

- 2. Write for 2 minutes a day describing one positive experience you had over the past 24 hours. This is a strategy to help transform you from a task-based thinker, to a meaning based thinker who scans the world for meaning instead of endless to-dos. This dramatically increases work happiness.

- 3. Exercise for 10 minutes a day. This trains your brain to believe your behavior matters, which causes a cascade of success throughout the rest of the day.

- 4. Meditate for 2 minutes, focusing on your breath going in and out. This will help you undo the negative effects of multitasking. Research shows you get multiple tasks done faster if you do them one at a time. It also decreases stress and raises happiness.

- 5. Write one, quick email first thing in the morning thanking or praising a member on your team. This significantly increases your feeling of social support, which in my study at Harvard was the largest predictor of happiness for the students.

- TAKE OUR 7-STEP HAPPINESS MASTERY SYSTEM and our 21-DAY HAPPINESS WORKOUT & KICKSTART from The Healing Academy!

PRACTICE THE 7 SPIRITUAL LAWS AND LAWS OF ATTRACTION

- The law of pure potentiality: Practice non-judgment. "Today I shall judge nothing that occurs, and throughout the day I shall remind myself not to judge."

- The law of giving: Give a gift to whoever you encounter, it could be anything. It doesn't have to be material, it could be as small as a compliment, a smile, or a hug. Those are all giving actions. "Today I will give something to everyone I come in contact with, and so I will begin the process of circulating joy, wealth, and affluence in my life and in the life of others."

- The law of "karma" or cause and effect: Witness the choices you make at each moment. "By witnessing my choices, I bring them to my conscious awareness, and I know that the best way to prepare for any moment in the future is to be fully conscious in the present."

- The law of least effort: Practice acceptance. Accept people, situations, and events as they occur. Be like a stream flowing with the current, and not like the rock straining against it. "Today I will not struggle against the whole universe by struggling against this moment. My acceptance is total and complete. I accept things as they are in this moment, as I wish they were."

- The law of intention and desire: Refuse to allow obstacles to consume and dissipate the quality of attention in the present moment. "I will remind myself to practice present-moment awareness in all my actions. I will accept the present as it is, and manifest the future through my deepest, most cherished intentions and desires."

- The law of detachment: Commit to detachment, to allow yourself and those around you to be as they are. "Today I will not rigidly impose my idea of how things should be. I will not force solutions on problems, thereby creating new problems. I will participate in everything with detached involvement."

- The law of "dharma" or purpose in life: Ask yourself, How can I serve? How can I help? How can I put my physical body to work? "When I express m y unique talents and express them in the service of humanity, I lose track of time and create abundance in my life as well as the lives of others."

- https://chopra.com/articles/the-7-spiritual-laws-of-success

- https://www.youtube.com/watch?v=Ny7G7AjtB10

- It doesn't have to be spiritual, but more a practice to bring a "Higher Power" – whatever you define it as into your life. Go Deep- Know Thyself: Steps? Know to whom you are speaking. …Thank him. …Ask for God's will. …Say what you need. …Ask for forgiveness. …Pray with a friend. …Pray the Word. …Memorize Scripture.

- https://www.ted.com/talks/rick_warren_on_a_life_of_purpose?language=en

- https://www.youtube.com/watch?v=7SJCDLHyeqk

- https://www.youtube.com/watch?v=_IDlvrHIZ4M

- Forgiveness: I believe the key to letting go of past trauma, resentment, anger, self-pity and other negative baggage is to learn how to forgive yourself and forgive others for perceived or real harms done. Steps: See forgiveness as a gift to you, not a gift to someone else. …Stop ruminating on negative feelings. …Identify your experience of the grudge. …Consider the impact holding on to the grudge has on you. …Ask yourself what you really need to do this. …Acknowledge that it happened. …Forgiveness is a process.

- Intentionally consecrate the time.

- Wake up just 20 minutes before the rest of your family does; or if you're a night owl, stay up a little longer than everyone else.

- Treat your shower like a fortress of solitude. …

- Do your daily run or workout in silence. …

- Commute to work in silence.

- https://www.artofmanliness.com/articles/spiritual-disciplines-solitude-silence/

- Keep a Gratitude journal and add to it everyday.

- Tell someone you love them and how much you appreciate them.

- Notice the beauty in nature each day.

- Nurture the friendships you have, good friends don't come along every day.

- Smile more often.

- Watch inspiring videos that will remind you of the good in the world.

- https://www.lifehack.org/articles/communication/40-simple-ways-practice-gratitude.html

- https://www.ted.com/talks/david_steindl_rast_want_to_be_happy_be_grateful?language=en

- https://www.ted.com/playlists/206/give_thanks

- 3 Steps to Define Success on Your Own Terms

- Success has ups and downs. Facing your fears is the key to happiness. And real success involves defining it on your own terms. The need for a universal definition of success is what constantly keeps us in a state of lack. Finding true success requires honoring the parts of you that are different than everyone else.

- 1. Define YOURSELF on your own terms. 2. Dare to be great. 3. Work for it. BUT, most importantly, know that success has nothing to do with the acquisition of external things and a big life, but rather in the quality of our relationships and happiness in life. Happiness comes before success and must be our priority. You can have it all, but happiness comes first!

- https://www.ted.com/talks/alain_de_botton_a_kinder_gentler_philosophy_of_success?language=en

- https://www.ted.com/talks/richard_st_john_s_8_secrets_of_success?language=en

- https://www.youtube.com/watch?v=McGlwCOL_ww

- More and more people are looking to reconnect themselves with nature and taking a step back from technology and the digital world to get in touch with mother earth. There is a holistic appeal to living off the land, cultivating and growing your own food where possible, generating your own energy and making a conscious effort to spend some time away from the computer, phone or television screens.

- Many Americans are looking to get back to nature because it's a healthier lifestyle option. It is not only more friendly for the environment, but eating fresh food, spending more time outdoors and being active can do wonders for an individual's health.

- Try these amazing ways to get into nature:

- Explore the great outdoors in your state, Plan a beach trip and make a difference Get out in the garden Hit the trails Look for a national or state park Walk in the forest, in a beautiful field, in an arboretum, or just someplace beautiful and outdoors. Go camping and watch the stars and planets in the night sky. Watch the universe through a telescope. Go horseback riding on a natural trail or on the beach, take an incredible adventure away in nature's way and background. Grow a garden, if you live in a city, walk in a park on the dirt barefoot and reconnect, go the mountains and breathe the mountain air, observe and study beautiful plants, gardens, trees, animals, insects – everything in God's backyard. Enjoy the natural beauty and breathe deeply and often with gratitude! Buy national geographic magazine, watch shows on nature. This is both necessary and a beautiful way to touch those things that are deeper

- Life is all about discovering your purpose in life and finding the meaning that makes your life worth living. That is the journey without a destination.

- 10 Life Purpose Tips to Help You Find Your Passion

- April 19, 2019 by Jack Canfield 21 Comments

- If you want to be fulfilled, happy, content, and experience inner peace and ultimate fulfillment, it's critical that you learn how to find your passion and life purpose. Without a life purpose as the compass to guide you, your goals and action plans may not ultimately fulfill you. 1. Explore the Things You Love To Do & What Comes Easy to You2. Ask Yourself What Qualities You Enjoy Expressing the Most in the World 3. Create a Life Purpose Statement4. Follow Your Inner Guidance (What Is Your Heart Telling You?) 5. Be Clear About Your Life Purpose 6. Conduct a Passion Test Great Resources:

- https://www.youtube.com/watch?v=z8XECSIoEgE

- https://www.youtube.com/watch?v=z8XECSIoEgE

- https://www.youtube.com/watch?v=z8XECSIoEgE

- https://www.youtube.com/watch?v=z8XECSIoEgE

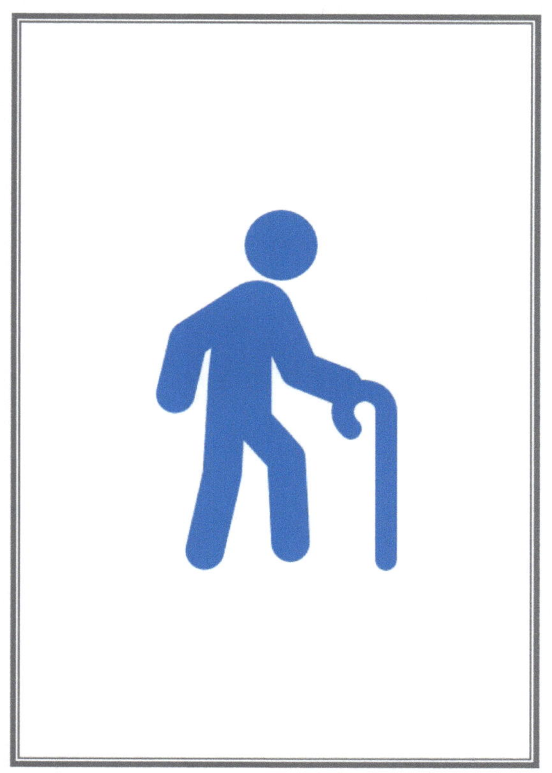

- As we know, the 100+ age group, "the centenarians," are the fastest growing age group north of 85. In the next decade, the number of centenarians is expected to nearly double.

- But, living to 100 and past, while amazing to witness, comes with many challenges. Aging diseases like Alzheimer's and Dementia are on the rise, as are many other age-related end of life diseases like cancer, cardiovascular, pulmonary, diabetes, and general decline of normal bodily functions, including mobility. While science is keeping us alive longer, it can also prolong the agony of aging and long-term suffering and pain. So, while living to a ripe, old age is a noble pursuit and wish for many, quality of life is a major consideration for those seeking to stay alive longer!

- We can live longer than ever by changing the way we process our lives.

- Blue Zones, science, technology, and practice have found formulas to lengthen and increase the quality of our lives

- Diet, exercise, nutrition, lots of great new habits and rituals can change the quality and quantity of our life

- We can live to be happy, joyous and free from the things that make us miserable, unhealthy, and less than the optimal human beings.

- Focus on experiences, relationships, and quality of your life if you want to live happily and longer: It's a scientific fact.

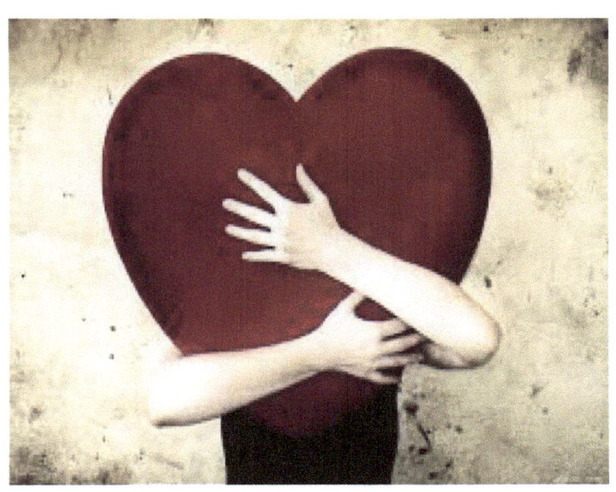

- THE HEALING ACADEMY (url)/facebook group)
- Healing from Toxic Parents
- Happiness Mastery System
- 21-Day Happiness Challenge
- Making Love Work
- Making Life Work
- Spiritual Journey
- Mindfulness & Meditation
- All my e-books

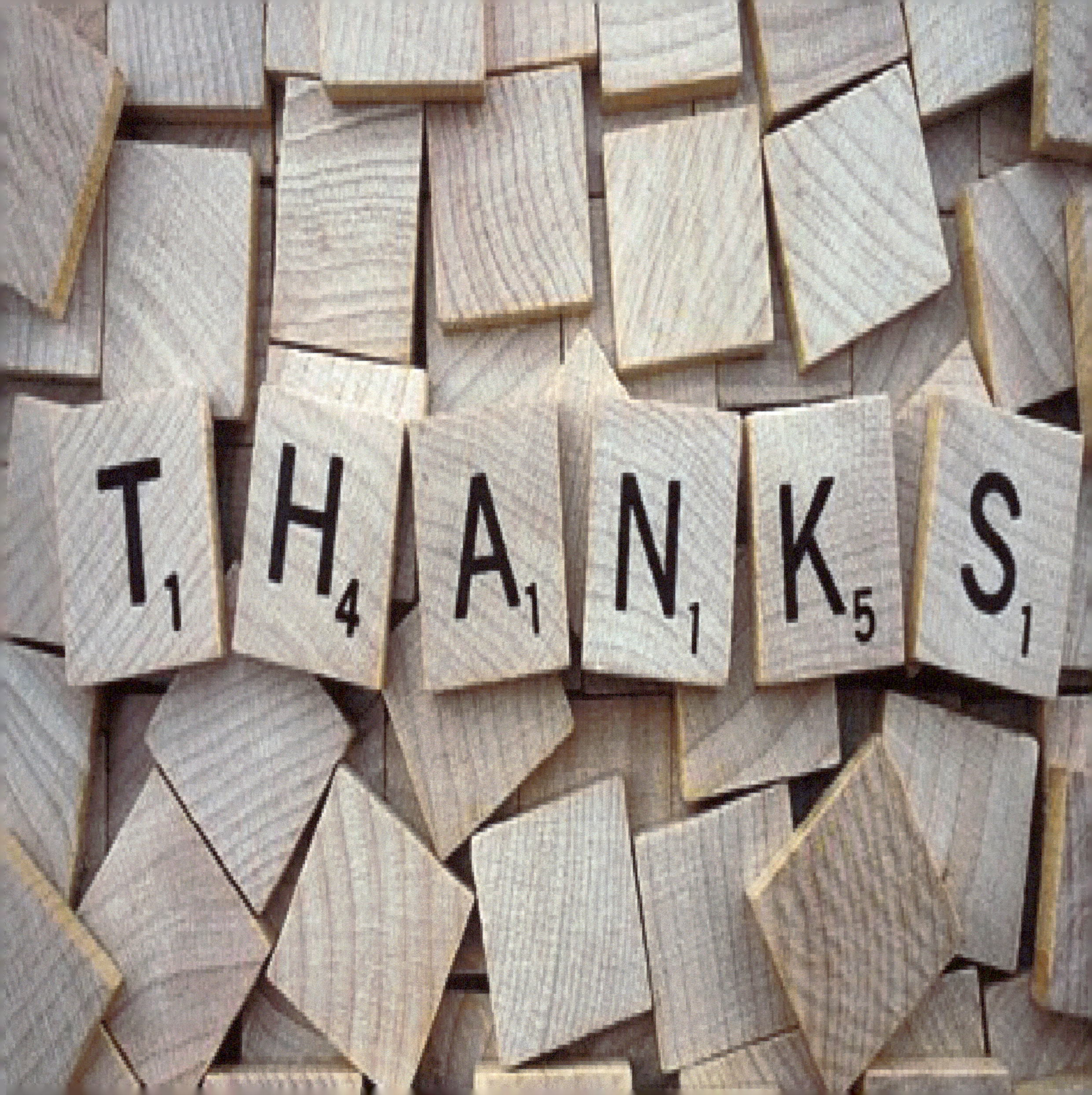
THANKS